Ketogenic Diet
For
Ultimate Weight Loss –
Lose Belly Fat Fast

Steven Ballinger

D1057641

Table of Contents

1: What is Ketogenic Diet and How Does it Work?

A diet that is high in fats, sufficient in proteins and low in carbs is known as the ketogenic diet. This began as a way to treat children who have refractory epilepsy, but it has also emerged as a way for adults to lose weight.

This diet makes the body consume fat instead of carbohydrates. In a normal diet, the body converts carbs from food into glucose and then sends it throughout the body, where it is very important for brain function.

However, when a diet has almost no carbs, the liver turns fat into ketone bodies and fatty acids. The ketone bodies move into the brain and provide energy in the place of glucose.

As the number of ketone bodies increases in the blood, the body enters ketosis, a state in which epileptic seizures happen less frequently. However, those who are not epileptic but simply want to lose weight can use this diet as well.

The original ketogenic diet had a 4:1 ratio of fat to the combination of carbs and protein. The easiest way to do this is to eliminate such carb-heavy foods, such as pasta, bread, sugar, grains and starchy vegetables or fruits. Instead, people eat foods that are higher in fat, such as nuts, as well as adding butter and cream to what they consume.

The ketogenic diet emerged in the 1920s, but the popularity of drugs that fight convulsions caused its popularity to decline. However, when Hollywood producer Jim Abrahams had a son who had epilepsy, the diet controlled the seizures.

Abrahams set up the Charlie Foundation so that others could find out about the diet, with publicity on news programs and a television movie that starred Meryl Streep. As with any dietary change, the ketogenic diet can lead to adverse effects, and in about a third of those who try it, constipation occurs. However, ensuring that you take in enough liquids keeps this from happening in most cases.

For those who are interested in weight loss only (rather than seizure management), the cyclical ketogenic diet is ideal. The most common way to follow this is to eat according to a ketogenic plan from Monday through Friday, working out three times.

On the weekends, you add carbs back into your diet and keep exercise at a minimum. The reason that this works is that the added carbs over the weekend help your body store some energy for the coming week, maintaining an adequate strength level for the workouts, and keeping your body out of what is called "starvation mode," where weight loss comes to a crawl.

The low calorie intake on the weekdays can lead your body into that sort of metabolic hibernation, so adding carbs back in two days a week keeps your body from shutting weight loss down. Having carbs on the weekends also means that it is easier to stay motivated, because you know you have the two days of carbs coming soon.

When you start out with this sort of diet, the best way to start is with an introductory phase of 10 to 14 days. For this entire time, pursue a diet low in carbs so that your body enters ketosis. Then, after those two weeks, you enter the five days/two days cycle of eating according to the cyclical diet.

You will notice several benefits after you have been on the cyclical diet for a week or so. It takes the body a while to adjust to major changes like this, and initially your body will miss the carbs, leading to cravings. One of these is that your appetite will actually go down. Hunger is often one of the primary reasons why diets go by the wayside.

People hate the miserable feeling of being hungry all the time, and they go back to the way they were eating. When you eat low carb, though, your body adjusts, and your appetite goes down. As a result, your caloric consumption goes down as well.

Another benefit is that diets that reduce carbs cause greater weight loss at a faster rate. This is true for several reasons.

First reason has to do with the fact that low carb diets send extra water out of the body. These diets tend to reduce insulin levels, allowing kidneys to expel extra sodium, and weight loss jump starts in the first week or so.

The only reason why these diets fail is that people tend to go back to their old habits after they lose a little bit of weight. This is why most nutritionists suggest considering this new way of eating as a lifestyle rather than a temporary diet.

The second reason is that those who follow low carb diets lose their fat from their abdominal cavity. This is referred to visceral fat, and it forms near the organs. People with more fat in those areas have greater resistance to insulin and higher levels of inflammation.

Many researchers believe that this type of fat is one of the main causes of metabolic difficulties throughout North America and Europe. Low carb diets tend to eliminate this visceral fat, leading to lower level type 2 diabetes and cardiac disease.

Finally, low carb diets also tend to lower blood pressure, eliminating the problems that come from hypertension (elevated blood pressure). Such conditions as stroke, kidney failure, cardiac disease and other conditions are much more likely when your blood pressure is higher.

In general terms, the ketogenic diet has shown major benefits, not just in terms of weight loss but also in other areas of people's health.

Before you start any major change in your diet or lifestyle, you need to talk to your physician to make sure that it is right for you, but the vast majority of people who have gone to a cyclical ketogenic diet report only positive outcomes.

Combining this diet with an exercise regimen is the best way to see the results you want in terms of weight loss, improved health and overall wellness.

The sooner you start making some of these changes to your lifestyle, the sooner you will reap the benefits!

2: Ketogenic Diet for Weight Loss

If you are pursuing the ketogenic diet as a way to lose weight, one of the most common sources of frustration is likely to be that your sweet tooth isn't getting the satisfaction it craves. This is going to be the case in just about any diet, but the fact is, the ketogenic diet involves eliminating most or all carbohydrates from your diet.

The cyclical ketogenic diet involves adding fats and cutting carbs five days and then adding carbs back in the other two days. As long as you exercise three times during those five days, you will still lose weight.

However, if you cheat by gratifying your sweet tooth during the other five days, you are going to fail. Here are some ways you can make the ketogenic diet work for weight loss by embracing the cycle and finding ways to satisfy your sweet tooth without the carbs.

Let's face it - if you love sweet foods, the idea of cutting carbs out can be downright scary. With some conventional diets, especially those that focus on cutting out fats, a common tactic is to replace, say, your bowl of ice cream with a bowl of fruit.

However, high sugar fruits like pineapples are also on the forbidden list with a ketogenic diet. While you can have berries, these might not be what you were thinking of when you thought that losing weight would be a good idea. One piece of good news is that the longer you can last on a low carb diet, the less your body will demand sugar.

Just as with any addictive substance, going through withdrawal from sugar is initially a process that your body will object to. However, as time goes by, your body will overcome its addiction to sugar, and you will see more consistent blood glucose levels. Also, the foods you eat on your new diet will start tasting sweeter, because your taste buds will adjust to the range of flavors that you are taking in.

You might even become someone who stops looking forward to a slice of cake or a couple of cookies after dinner altogether. However, while you're waiting for your body to stop craving for sugar, or if you're not one of those people who ends up leaving sugar behind, here are some tips to help you in the meantime.

Sugar Free Foods and Beverages

Quite a few of the most popular sodas and other treats, such as Jell-O or ice cream, come in sugar free varieties. Some of this is due to the high number of diabetics in the population, whose numbers have created significant demand for alternative sources of sweetness. If you are in the initial phases of your ketogenic diet, choose sodas that lack caffeine as well, such as Sprite Zero or Fresca rather than a diet cola.

Artificial Sweeteners

There are quite a few different sugar substitutes, such as Sweet N Low and Equal. However, the best one that maintains flavor across temperatures and works well in cooking applications is Splenda. It also lacks some of the health risks that the other two sugar substitutes have been associated with. If you purchase Splenda in granulated form, you can add it to your tea or coffee and use it when you cook. You can even dash some of it onto the food that you want to sweeten.

Low Carb Foods

Thanks to the popularity of the Atkins and South Beach diets, both of which involve the elimination of carbs from the diet, there are many different food products that are friendly to the ketogenic diet.

Snack bars and cookies are available in a low carb format that you can eat, even on your days when you are avoiding carbs. These products are manufactured for people who are pursuing a diet low in carbs, and the number of carbs in each snack appears on the packaging, giving you the tools you need to manage your diet.

Berries

Like we said earlier, you can have berries on the days when you're supposed to be limiting just about all of the carbs from your diet. After all, berries aren't just low in carbs; they're also high in antioxidants and other nutrients that your body needs in order to maintain health.

They add a bit of sweetness to your food, but they don't make your blood sugar spike. Make sure that you keep an eye on your portions and add those carbs to your daily count.

There are a couple of misconceptions that people have associated with the ketogenic diet for weight loss. One of these is that the higher fat content associated with this diet leads to heart attacks. If you are eating a diet with a lot of carbs as well as fat, your body holds onto that fat, blocking arteries and boosting the overall fat ratio in the body.

This is what leads to cardiac arrest as well as a number of other complications. However, when you have achieved ketosis, your body gets its energy primarily from fat, which means that it won't store the fat - it will burn it instead. Another misconception is that diets low-in-carbs are bad for your kidneys. It is true that some people who have renal issues get the advice to eat a diet lower in protein. However, the misconception comes from the fact that many people believe that all low carb diets are high in protein.

The ketogenic diet, while high in fat, is not necessarily so high in protein. This means that your kidneys won't be getting the same stress they would be getting otherwise.

If you remember that the ketogenic diet is cyclical in nature, with five low or no-carb days followed by two days in which you can consume carbs, then finding your way to weight loss will be easier. You'll have the upcoming incentive of extra carbs on the weekend to keep you following the plan during the week. Trying the suggestions in this article will help you succeed in the challenge of losing weight.

3: Using Ketogenic Diet to Lose Belly Fat Fast!

If you're interested in losing weight, then you no doubt know the magic number for weight loss: to lose a pound of mass, you have to burn 3,500 more calories than you take in.

However, if you look around, not everyone appears to be carrying their weight the same way. Some of this comes from genetics, and some of this comes from lifestyle choices. Some people have a body type that amasses fat in the belly area, while others take fat on more uniformly across their bodies.

While you can't fight your genes, you can make the right lifestyle choices when it comes to the fat that you take in, and starting a ketogenic diet is one of the best choices you can make when it comes to removing your belly fat quickly.

It is important to realize that hormones tell our body what to do with the food that comes in. One of the most important hormones in this area is insulin. When you take in glucose, your body releases insulin, and any carbohydrates that you consume break down into glucose.

The more glucose you have in your bloodstream, the more insulin your body sets loose. Your body has to deal with glucose, because if the levels get too high, glucose becomes a toxin. As a result, your liver and muscles can store it, or your body can burn it through metabolic processes, or you can store it as fat.

Because you're converting your body to ketosis, though, you won't burn glucose - but fat instead. You're going to bring your carb consumption down close to zero, which means that the insulin hormone won't be circulating through your blood telling your body to shove fat into a place you don't want it. Instead, you'll be burning it.

This is why the ketogenic diet is one of the best ways to shed belly fat. Any low carb diet limits the glucose you're taking in, keeping you from spiking in glucose (and then spiking in insulin, and then storing glucose as fat).

A recent discovery of how insulin works makes it simple to understand why so many people in the West have issues with weight. So many meals have more than 100 grams of carbohydrates that digest quickly and then absorb as fat.

Pizza, sandwich bread, hamburger buns, noodles, cereals, and drinks with sugar all tell your body to send insulin around the body. These foods all contain processed carbohydrates. Because the body has an easier time breaking these down, the glucose inside hits our bloodstream more quickly and in greater volume than fruits and vegetables - even the starchy and sugary ones.

If you drink a 20 ounce bottle of Coke or Sprite, you are taking in as much sugar as you would by eating nine cups of strawberries. Remember that glucose is ultimately toxic if the levels get to high, so your body has to figure out what to do with it.

When you exercise, you use the glucose that is in your muscles and then liver. If those areas have little or no glucose left, what you take in goes to those repositories before it goes to fat.

The average active person only needs 150 grams of carbohydrates each day to keep full levels of glycogen in the liver and muscles. In the West, the average person takes in about 300 grams of carbohydrates on a daily basis. Their activity levels are low (no, Facebooking doesn't count as exercise).

This means that each meal adds more glucose into your fat storage area. Also, every meal is followed by the introduction of a hormone (insulin) that hinders you from burning fat as energy. Wonder why it's so hard to lose weight?

You may also have read about the increasing number of cases of type 2 diabetes among Western societies. This increase is a direct consequence of the ways our diet influences our insulin.

If you have habitually eaten a high carb diet, you have likely built up some degree of insulin resistance. You feel lethargic, gain weight and are at risk of type 2 diabetes. The good news is that this is easy to turn around with a ketogenic diet.

Another hormone that is important to understand when you are thinking about burning belly fat is cortisol. This is the hormone that your body uses to signal the need to release the energy that is being stored inside fat cells.

Your cortisol levels are highest first thing in the morning, but any time your body has stress that is physical or mental, cortisol enters the system as well. Balanced cortisol levels are a good thing.

However, because of the high levels of stress that are a part of modern life for too many of us, it is easy for cortisol levels to get out of control. When your cortisol levels are too high, your body will fight fat loss, and you will gain more weight.

If there is a layer of fat on your belly that you just cannot lose, no matter how hard you exercise or how well you diet, your cortisol levels are probably too high.

So how does the ketogenic diet interact with these hormones? The magic word here is leptin. This is the hormone that tells you to stop eating because you are full. Your body sends out a lot of leptin when you take in proteins and fats and a little when you take in carbohydrates.

Think about it. Would you be able to eat more slices of bacon or French toast sticks? Which would make you feel full (or even a little green at the gills) faster? The bacon will make you feel full sooner, and you'll feel full longer.

This is why so many healthy snacks for weight loss have protein in them, because they signal your body to send out leptin so you don't go back to the pantry for chips after you have your snack.

Staying away from carbs and sticking with high protein and high fat meals, you stop eating sooner, your blood glucose levels stay manageable, and that belly fat starts to fall away, particularly if you stick with a regular exercise regimen.

4: Low Carb Recipes

It's one thing to commit to eat a low carb diet as part of your ketogenic weight loss plan. It's another to live that way on a day to day basis, because it's a challenge to prepare meals that suit the requirements.

Most of the foods that are easy to grab and eat are high in carbs. Want a sandwich? That bread you put on there will blow your carb numbers for the day. The same goes for the majority of those chips you want to snack on.

Having some recipes in your arsenal will help you prepare for ketogenic eating. Take a look at some of these ideas - you can cook several meals on one day and then freeze them for your busy days in the middle of the week.

Breakfast Recipe: Three Cheese Quiche

Love eggs and cheese? You can have plenty of these on the ketogenic diet. Traditional quiches have a crust (which would have too many carbs), but this one does not. Even so, it's fluffy, light and tall when you make it right.

Preparation time: 15 minutes

Cooking time: 45 minutes to bake plus time to stand and cool

Ingredients:

7 eggs
5 egg yolks
1 cup half and half
1 cup heavy whipping cream
3/4 cup sharp cheddar cheese, shredded and divided
1/2 cup Swiss cheese, shredded
1 cup part skim mozzarella cheese, shredded
2 tablespoons oil packed sun dried tomatoes, finely chopped
1 1/2 teaspoons salt free seasoning
1/4 teaspoon dried basil

Nutritional Information

If you eat one piece, you are taking in 449 calories, 37 grams of fat (21 of those are saturated), 524 mg of cholesterol, 316 mg of sodium, a measly 5 grams of carbohydrates and 22 grams of protein.

Instructions

Preheat the oven to 350 degrees. Combine the yolks, eggs, half and half, whipping cream, 1/2 cup of cheddar cheese, all the other cheeses, basil, seasoning and tomatoes. Pour the mixture into a nine inch deep dish pie plate that you have already greased. Sprinkle the rest of the cheddar cheese on top. Bake for 45 minutes or until you can slide a knife in near the middle and have it come out clean. Before cutting, allow it to stand for at least 10 minutes. You will get six servings from this recipe.

Lunch Recipe: BLT Salad

One of the classic sandwiches in American cuisine is the BLT (bacon, lettuce and tomato). Get the bread out of the equation by converting this into a salad. With the tomato and chive dressing in this recipe, you get a boost of flavor as well as some extra Vitamin C - without the carbs that come with those two big slices of bread.

Preparation Time: 25 minutes of active work

Ingredients:

1 cup whole wheat bread, cubed
2 teaspoons extra virgin olive oil
3 slices center cut bacon, cooked thoroughly and crumbled
4 medium tomatoes, divided
2 tablespoons chives, minced
3 tablespoons low fat mayonnaise

2 teaspoons distilled white vinegar
1/4 teaspoon garlic powder
5 cups hearts of romaine lettuce, chopped
Pepper to taste

Nutritional Information

Each serving gives you 151 calories, 6 grams of fat
(1 saturated gram), 5 milligrams of cholesterol, 20
grams of carbs (0 grams of added sugar), 4 grams
of fiber, 5 grams of protein, 306 milligrams of
sodium and 555 milligrams of potassium. You also
get 110 percent of your daily value of Vitamin A
and 60 percent of your daily value of Vitamin C, as
well as almost a third of your daily value of folate.

Instructions

Preheat the oven to 350 degrees. Toss the bread in
with the oil, and then spread across a baking sheet.
Turn the bread once while you're baking it, leaving
it in the oven until it turns golden brown, or for 15
or 20 minutes. Cut one of the tomatoes in half.

Shred both halves with a box grater, using the big
holes. Toss the skin away. Add the chives,
mayonnaise, garlic powder, vinegar and pepper,
whisking the combination to blend. Chop the other
tomatoes, and add them with the croutons and

romaine to your bowl. Toss the whole thing to provide an even coat. Sprinkle the bacon over the top.

Low Carb Dinner: Pork Chops with Blackberry Sauce

If you think that ketogenic living will mean salad after salad, you have another thing coming. The delicious flavors of pork and blackberry in this recipe are so good that you just might make this meal during one of the days when you can eat the carbs that you want. Avoid the temptation to serve these with legumes; instead, serve with some steamed spinach with butter to get the results that you want.

Ingredients:

4 bone in pork loin chops (7 oz. each)
1/4 cup seedless blackberry spreadable fruit
3 teaspoons ketchup
1/4 teaspoon garlic, minced
1/4 teaspoon mustard
1/4 teaspoon cornstarch
1 tablespoon steak sauce

Nutritional Information

If you have one pork chop with two tablespoons of sauce on it, you'll have 261 calories, 8 grams of fat (3 of them saturated), 86 milligrams of cholesterol, 279 milligrams of sodium, 14 grams of carbs and 30 grams of protein.

Instructions

Broil the pork chops for about five minutes on each side, until your meat thermometer shows 145 degrees. Then set aside to stand for five minutes before plating. While they're broiling, combine the mustard, garlic, ketchup and spreadable fruit in a small saucepan. Place on the stove before bringing to a boil. Add the steak sauce and cornstarch until smooth, and then stir into the pan. Bring to a boil again, stirring and cooking for two minutes until thickened. Total yield is four servings.

Dessert: Sugar Free Coconut Macaroons

These are simple to make, with just a few ingredients and taking only 15 minutes to cook.

Ingredients:

2 tablespoons water
2 cups unsweetened coconut, shredded
4 egg whites

1 teaspoon vanilla extract
1 cup sugar substitute, such as liquid Splenda

Nutritional Information

Every cookie has just a gram of carbohydrates to go along with 76 calories, 2 grams of fiber and 2 grams of protein.

Instructions

Preheat the oven to 375 degrees. Line a baking sheet with parchment paper. Measure out the egg whites, adding water if necessary to bring the level of 1/2 cup. Add the liquid sweetener and vanilla with additional water, ending up with a total of two tablespoons of sweetener and water. If you are using a powdered sweetener instead, add it to the coconut.

Mix all of the ingredients together. Allow it to set for a couple of minutes. Roll the mixture into balls that are about an inch in diameter, or a little larger. Flatten slightly and then place them on the baking sheet, giving a half inch or space between each cookie.

Reduce the temperature to 325 degrees and then bake the cookies for approximately 15 minutes.

Start looking at them after about 10 minutes, though. They should look golden brown underneath while just barely brown on the top. On average, this recipe yields about 14 cookies.

5: Understanding Ketosis

Ketogenic diet is based on the principal of ketosis. Ketosis is basically a state where the body after being starved of glucose starts to burn fat. The metabolism of the fat releases compounds called ketones. Ketones have the added advantage of being used for energy purposes as well as for powering up the brain.

Other organs like the heart also have the need for some certain specific ketone molecules. Ketogenic diet has been used for medical reason in the treatment of extreme epilepsy in children. The increased ketone levels in the brain help control epileptic attacks.

The ketogenic diet is also used for weight loss purposes because of its fat burning properties. Certain negative effects may occur during the transition of the body from its normal glucose burning state to ketosis. Weakness, fatigue, headaches and light headedness are some of the symptoms that may manifest. They should last just a week or so after starting the ketogenic diet.

Research has shown that besides epilepsy and weight loss the ketogenic diet has also proven helpful in Type 2 Diabetes and Cardiovascular ailments.

Now let's take a look at the different dietary components of the ketogenic diet.

Carbohydrate

The amount of carbohydrate consumed by the individual depends on one's activity level and metabolism. Essentially one would consume anywhere between 50 to 60 grams of net carbohydrate a day. But a person with a healthy metabolism may consume up to 100 grams and still remain in ketosis. Older people with slow metabolism may be restricted to below 30 grams per day.

Protein

As you start off with ketogenic diet you will find that the amount of protein intake won't be as important as in the later stages. The body slowly adapts and learns to convert protein into glucose efficiently and hence may be thrown out of ketosis. So with time you must learn to monitor the amount of protein you consume and determine if it is messing with ketosis.

Fat

The amount of fat to be consumed depends on the actual consumption of proteins and carbohydrates during the diet. It is also determined by the activity rate and how fast they are losing weight. Essentially about 60 to 80 percent of you total calories should come from fat. It can even be up to 90 percent during the treatment of epilepsy.

The type of fats to be consumed is also very important for maintain good health. People on the ketogenic diet are advised to steer clear of fats with high levels of polyunsaturated fats. Salad dressing, mayonnaise etc. are some examples.

Fats which have high quantities of triglycerides, like coconut oil are recommended as these can be easily broken down into ketones by our body. Normally a person on a ketogenic diet will consume large quantities of saturated and monounsaturated fats like cheese, butter, olive oil etc.

You can easily lose your unwanted belly fat if you follow the above mentioned points while embarking upon a ketogenic diet. A single day's meal would be similar to the one mentioned below:

Breakfast

Peanut butter Cereal (Flax)
A quarter cup of blueberries along with the cereal

Lunch

Salad with romaine lettuce
avocado and chicken accompanied by vinaigrette
dressing.

Snack

A quarter cup of almonds

Dinner

Pan fried or grilled steak
Green beans
Mushrooms and peppers with herbs and wine

Calories can be easily varied by adding or
subtracting fat or proteins of the diet. Another
suggestion would be to follow the following meal
plan for 7 days. From Monday to Wednesday you
can have Chorizo Breakfast Casserole, for lunch go
for the Mexican Spinach Casserole and for dinner
eat a Caveman Chili. You can easily find the

recipes online. Modify the dishes according to your calorie needs.

For the next two days change your dinner to a Creamy Cheesy Sandwich and Chicken. For the weekend we make it grand and start off the day with a Bacon Open Weave Sandwich, followed by a Taco Salad for lunch and for dinner go for a Meatza, which is like a pizza but uses ground beef for its base. Again all meal proportions should be governed by your metabolic requirements and your activity rate.

It normally takes about 2-3 weeks for the actual ketosis to begin and the weightless to show. Sometime if you feel that you are not reaching ketosis then subtle tweaks in your diet can be done to remedy this. Some people measure their ketone levels while on the diet.

If you are getting what you want and are losing weight steadily this practice is not necessary. But if you feel that you are not achieving your target you can have a look at your blood ketone levels. Ideally while on the diet they should hover around the .5 mmol/L to 3 mmol/L mark.

Also special Ketostixs are available in the market which can help measure the amount of acetone in our urine. Acetone is a ketone which is discarded by the body through urine and can help given an estimate on the ketone levels present in our system. The more the acetone the more the stick will burn.

The Ketogenic diet is a proven way to lose weight and has added health benefits. New research has shown it aids in cases where the patient is suffering from neurological disorders other than Epilepsy, Acne and Certain types of cancer.

The Ketogenic succeeds where the Atkins diet fails. People on the Atkins diet end up adding more carbohydrate than necessary and their bodies fall out of ketosis. Also the ketogenic diet takes into account the chance that overdue course of time the proteins will also start getting converted to glucose thus disrupting ketosis.

Some people skeptical of the ketogenic diet may argue that not enough glucose is being provided for sustenance. The fact to be pointed out is that the measured amounts of carbohydrates and proteins being consumed make up for any specific glucose requirements the body must have. Hence the ketogenic diet is completely safe and can be adopted to lose unwanted fat from problems areas like you tummy.

6: Fruits and Vegetables with Low Carbs

Many people think that simply adding a regimen of fruits and vegetables to their diet will make the pounds melt off. It's true that pineapple is a more nutritious snack than potato chips, but pineapple has a lot of calories too, in the form of fructose (the sugar that is found in fruits).

There are even some vegetables that are fairly high in carbs, which can be a trap for people trying to lose weight with a low carb diet. This section contains a list of some of the more common low carb fruits and vegetables, in rough order from lowest to highest in terms of carbs per serving.

However, all of the foods on this list are low in carbs and will work well on a ketogenic diet.

Low Carb Vegetables

Alfalfa sprouts

Throwing these on top of a salad gives you a bit more fiber without adding much at all in the way of starches or carbs. However, legumes with sprouts tend to have a little more in the way of carbs.

Greens

Fill your plate with spinach, chard, lettuce and other similar greens. You might have to add some other foods to provide enough flavor to make this a palatable option, but greens are basically roughage that also help you get some key nutrients, such as iron. You can eat as much of these as you want, because the caloric and carb input is minimal.

Hearty greens

These are things like kale, mustard greens and collard greens. There is a little more flavor with these dishes, but you also get some more carbs in the mix. Even so, though, you are still fine on the ketogenic index.
Herbs

These don't have to just be garnish on your plate, as basil, cilantro, thyme, rosemary and other herbs add a good bit of flavor to your meal. If having some more spinach just doesn't sound appetizing, throwing some of these herbs on top can make that meal look a lot more attractive.

Bok Choy

Also known as Pak Choi, or Chinese cabbage, this vegetable belongs in the brassica family with the other cabbages. There are fewer carbs in this variety than there are in the typical round cabbages you see in the grocery store.

Look for the dark leaves and the long white stalks. When it is in season, there is a smaller variety called Shanghai bok choy, or baby bok choy, that is more tender. Either way, this is a nutritious vegetable with minimal carbs.

Celery

This is a low carb vegetable that is quite versatile, usable in soups as well as a stand-alone snack, with cream cheese or peanut butter as an accompaniment. With some more flavor than some of the other vegetables on this list, celery is one of the more popular low carb vegetables.

Brussels sprouts

These are an acquired taste that often requires significant seasoning and butter to make it palatable. The good news is that butter and seasonings are two things that people on the ketogenic diet can have, so be creative with the way you prepare these veggies.

Snow peas

These are cool and crunchy when served raw, while retaining their crispy texture when you add them to a stir fry. The pleasant flavor makes this a favorite among ketogenic eaters.

Tomatoes

These red vegetables are bursting with flavor, as well as the nutrient lycopene, which has been proven to boost heart health. Low in carbs, tomatoes are a snack that you can sprinkle some pepper on after slicing into small wedges as part of a healthy snack.

Low Carb Fruits

You're going to have fewer choices when it comes to fruits than you will with vegetables, because all fruits contain fructose, a sugar that contributes to their sweet flavor. However, there are a number of fruits that you can incorporate into your diet. These appear roughly in order from lowest to highest in terms of carbohydrates.

Lemon/Lime

Obviously, you won't be cutting these up and eating them, but adding portions to drinks gives you some added flavor without adding much of anything to your carb count. If you're trying to drink more water, then adding a slice of one of these can make it a lot more palatable.

Raspberries

High in antioxidants, raspberries are a fairly tart fruit that nonetheless adds freshness to your plate. Blackberries and cranberries are actually good choices as well. All of these have a ton of fiber, minerals and vitamins, in addition to those antioxidants that promote better health, and may even keep you from developing heart disease and cancer as time goes by. There are some researchers that believe that these antioxidants even slow down the process of aging. It just takes a cup to give you your entire day's required portion of Vitamin C.

Strawberries

These have a little more sugar than the other berries, but unless you add whipped cream or syrup, you're not taking in too many carbs to make these a solid idea on the ketogenic diet.

Watermelon

Particularly popular in the summertime, watermelons are a great way to keep yourself hydrated while also getting the dietary fiber that fruit provides. You can't eat as much of these as you can the berries, because of the sugar involved, but you can add smaller portions to your plate.

Peaches and nectarines

These are about as high as you want to go in terms of sugars when you're on the ketogenic diet. Also in season during the summer, these are a great way to satisfy your sweet tooth without undoing the good of your ketogenic eating plan.

Remember that the best ketogenic diet is a cyclical one, so you can have the sugars you want on the weekends. Love grapefruits and plums? They have more sugar, but you can eat them on your two days of the ketogenic cycle. Use this shopping list as you head to the produce department each week to shop for your coming weight loss. If you can stick to these foods, you will make losing weight much easier!

7: Ketogenic Diet Menu for Diabetics

If you are already suffering from type 2 diabetes, your body has reached the point of resistance to insulin. Your body sends insulin out to the bloodstream as a response to your consumption of anything with sugar in it, but over time, you consumed enough glucose for your body to build up a resistance to this insulin, and it no longer can keep your glucose levels from becoming toxic.

That's why you have to have insulin in reserve and also need to have sugary snacks on hand just in case your sugar levels go down too far. It's not a great way to live, but the good news is that a ketogenic diet can help you find a more palatable quality of life. The key lies in planning your meals so that you eat the right things, and your blood sugar levels remain much more stable.

First, here's a good idea of what you shouldn't do. You want to keep steady levels of blood glucose and insulin, right? So don't take in any foods that are going to threaten that balance. If you look at the meal plans that the American diabetic Association has suggested, go back and take a look at the carbohydrates in each meal.

The guidelines that they have put out for you indicate that you can have between 60 and 75 grams of carbohydrates with each meal. Even if you're active, you only need 150 grams to stay fueled. Their plan would give you between 180 and 225 grams, well more than what you need. If you don't get much exercise, then you need closer to 100 than 150. If you're taking in 225, you're not doing yourself any favors.

You might be thinking that 50 or 75 grams too many really isn't that many. Let's take a look at the research. If you ingest 75 grams of carbohydrates in one meal, when you get up from the table, your blood sugar levels will sit at an average of 198 mg/dL. Now, let's look back at the recommended levels for that.

The maximum recommended post prandial (after eating) level is 170 mg/dL. It's kind of ironic that the American diabetic Association recommends a meal plan that sends your sugar about 30 points higher than the recommended level, but that's where things are.

Also, take a look at some of the staples that the American diabetic Association recommends. Potatoes and light yogurt often appear in their meal plans, but there are studies that show that either of these foods can send your insulin levels into a frenzy.

So why would this organization make flawed recommendations? It could be that the recommendation of a diet slightly higher in carbs is to cut down on the number of episodes with low blood sugar that you have.

These episodes can be fairly dangerous if you are on insulin. However, if you lower your carbs on a slow but steady basis, you will see results that are better. You can also reduce your medicine gradually as well, leaving the glucose merry-go-round behind.

So what kind of meals goes into a diabetic meal plan according to ketogenic principles? Remember that the emphasis is on proteins and fats. These types of meals help you manage your blood sugar more effectively.

The ketogenic diet helps you manage this more effectively. One typical meal might consist of 6 ounces of grilled salmon, with two cups of sautéed squash and two tablespoons of butter on the side.

Wrap that meal up with a cup of blackberries or a peach. Your total calories for that meal would be about 625, and your ratios of carbs to protein to fat would be roughly 15 to 25 to 60.

Based on the significant amount of research out there on the ways ketogenic diets can affect dietary health for diabetics (as well as non-diabetics), this is a ratio that would keep your blood sugar levels under 130 mg/dL, if not even lower.

Also, the delicious sirloin (and the yummy butter on the squash) would make you feel happy at the table and satisfy your hunger more effectively. These are factors that would help you keep your diet more faithfully, keeping your insulin and sugar levels stable and healthy.

Here's how a full day of ketogenic eating would look for a diabetic. For breakfast, haul some of that quiche out that you made over the weekend and put into the freezer. Cut yourself a slice, and pour yourself a cup of coffee with cream. You're looking at a meal under 500 calories with more than 70 percent fat and less than 5 percent from carbs.

So what about lunch? Steam a cup of broccoli, and add a tablespoon of butter. That's not all, though - you also get to have eight ounces of baked salmon, with two tablespoons of hollandaise sauce on top.

Add 1/2 cup of blueberries drizzled with an ounce of cream. You're less than 800 calories for the meal, about seven percent from carbs but almost 80 percent from fat.

Finish up your meals at the dinner table with a cup of cole slaw and a cup of steamed cauliflower with a tablespoon of (you guessed it) butter on it. Add six ounces of a low carb meatloaf recipe.

Your meal is under 900 calories, and your ratios (7% carb, 15% protein and 78% fat) are ideal for the ketogenic diet. Before you go to bed, have a glass of creamy chocolate milk. Your day has included fewer than 30 grams of carbs and just over 2000 calories.

Following these meal principles will help you avoid the complications of diabetes and keep your blood sugar and insulin levels more consistent. You'll be able to reduce your reliance on your medication, and over time you will feel better.

The issues with weight that led to your insulin resistance in the first place will ease, and you will find yourself craving carbs less and less. And who doesn't love a diet that lets you eat bacon? You'll want to talk to your doctor before beginning this program, but following this type of meal plan has worked wonders for many. With any luck, it can work wonders for you as well.

8: Ketogenic Diet for Aging

When it comes to the aging process, there are quite a few theories going around. Some have to do with genetics, while others focus on the damage that takes place in body tissues and cellular structures. Having the knowledge of some of these theories can make the benefits of ketogenic diet easier to understand.

Free Radicals and Aging

The role of free radicals in aging is the basis of one of the most commonly promulgated aging theory. On just about every wellness website, you can find mention of these things called "free radicals" as well as the solution for them, known as antioxidants.

Free radicals are molecules which are chemically reactive, and they are commonly known as reactive oxygen species, or ROS. These connect to cells, leading to inflammation and damage to proteins and genetic material in the cell's nucleus.

These free radicals are called "chemically reactive" because they are short on electron. They rove through cells looking for an electron to swipe from another molecule. The process through which this takes place is known as oxidation, and it leads to a sequence of damage.

When one electron gets stolen by a free radical, the victim molecule now is missing an electron, meaning that it is reactive too. It grabs an electron, and the vicious cycle continues. As time goes by, the damage increases, and the aging process speeds up.

According to this theory, the best way to stop this sort of damage and retard the process of aging is to boost the level of antioxidants in the body. Antioxidants work because they have an electron to give away. They neutralize the free radicals, stopping the chain of damage before it can really get started.

The majority of the free radicals in the body come from normal chemical reactions, like those that make energy inside our mitochondria. Other sources come from consuming a lot of polyunsaturated vegetable oils or smoking.

Not having enough antioxidants leads to an increased level of damage, which is why increasing antioxidant levels is so important in reversing the aging process.

Glycation and Aging

The theory that high blood sugars cause the aging process to accelerate centers around a process known as glycation. This involves excess glucose in the bloodstream binding to proteins that form the basis of our body tissues and cells.

As time goes by, these tissues form structures known as advanced glycation end products, or AGEs. These limit the efficiency of protein functions, to the point where proteins can no longer communicate or perform as necessary.

Such effects as atherosclerosis, nerve damage and vision loss, as well as complications associated with diabetes, are among the possibilities. Imagine pouring the syrup from a jar of maraschino cherries on your television remote, and then expecting the remote to perform its normal functions.

As blood sugar levels go up, glycation does as well. High fructose consumption appears to accelerate the process further -- perhaps as much as 10 times when compared to simple glucose in the blood.

The Ketogenic Diet and Aging

There are several ways in which ketogenic diets inhibit the aging process, which makes it popular in addition to its effectiveness in helping with weight loss.

First, ketogenic diets cut down on baseline sugar levels in the blood. In simple terms, this cuts down the glycation rate, meaning that those advanced glycation end products do not form as quickly. The damage to your proteins, then, takes much longer to occur.

A ketogenic diet also reduces your triglycerides, fatty acids that show up in the bloodstream. This might seem counterintuitive, because you are consuming more fats with this diet.

However, your body is learning to use the fat as fuel, so the fatty acids are being consumed by your body instead of sent into you bloodstream. When your triglyceride count is high, your body has the tendency to produce more advanced glycation end products.

When your body enters ketosis, you produce more mitochondrial glutathione. This is a crucial antioxidant that operates inside your mitochondria, which are a main staging ground for the work of free radicals.

One reason why this is so important is that many antioxidants that you consume orally have a hard time making it into the mitochondria, leaving the free radicals able to do a great deal more damage.

Ketogenic diets boosts your body's creation of uric acid and other powerful natural antioxidants. One reason why this is so important, whether you're talking about aging, neurological protection or weight loss, the stress that oxidants provide wreaks havoc in matters from the brain to many of the cells throughout the body.

Conditions like ALS, Parkinson's disease, Alzheimer's disease, stroke and traumatic brain injury all appear to feature oxidative stress as a potential cause.

Finally, ketogenic diets improve your body's ability to manage blood sugar levels and curb hunger. When you're eating less, you're cutting down on the oxidative damage that takes place inside your body, according to a number of research studies.

So how does a ketogenic diet help stop the aging process? There are mechanisms in most of the systems of the body that, based on existing research, appear to respond in a positive way to the changes that take place when the body enters ketosis, burning fats for energy instead of glucose.

When your blood sugar levels go down, so do the number of glycation end products, insulin levels in the blood and instances of inflammation. These three elements are closely connected with a wide variety of diseases that all contribute to earlier mortality.

In the final analysis, a ketogenic diet is a great way to cut your levels of insulin and blood sugar, which will increase your sense of well-being as well as your longevity.

While there are some side effects that show up in a percentage of the people who switch to this diet, current research indicates that, for most people, the side effects are manageable and do not outweigh the benefits of weight loss and a slower aging process.

Talk to your physician to see if a ketogenic diet is the right choice to help your own aging process slow down!

9: Ketogenic Diet for Brain Health

It's important to remember that the ketogenic diet actually creates a sensation of starvation, as the body changes over to the metabolic state known as ketosis. Instead of running on sugar, the body runs on fat -- specifically, the ketone bodies that your liver pulls out of fatty acids.

The three types of ketones are acetone, acetoacetate and BHB (beta hydroxybutyrate). When they enter the bloodstream, your brain and other organs snap them up and pull them into their mitochondria, using them for fuel. Extra ketones either go out through your urine (although acetone comes out through your breath).

When your brain pulls these ketones in, one of the effects appears to be protection against a number of brain diseases. So while this diet came about as a way to manage epilepsy, it has also shown promise as a way to shield the brain in several other ways.

So how does this work? One possible answer has to do with energy. Many neurological disorders share one commonality: insufficient production of energy. When metabolic stress occurs, ketones provide another source of energy to keep normal metabolism in brain cells up and running.

It appears that BHB may be more efficient than glucose, giving more energy for each unit of oxygen in use. Ketogenic diets also boost the numbers of mitochondria, known as the brain's energy factories. One recent study located an enhanced gene expression when it comes to encoding for energy metabolism within your hippocampus (the brain sector dedicated to memory and learning) as well as mitochondrial enzymes.

When brain diseases related to age strike, the cells in the hippocampus often degenerate, which leads to memory loss and cognitive issues. With a boost in the reserve of energy, neurons may gain the ability to fight of the stressors that normally kill those cells.

Another possible benefit of the ketogenic diet for the brain is that this eating plan may reduce the effects of one of the prime sources of stress on neurons. When cellular metabolism takes place, reactive oxygen is one of the by-products. This is not the same thing as oxygen - instead, these oxidants just have one electron.

As a result, they are more highly reactive, crashing into membranes and proteins. The more oxidants you have, the more your risk of stroke, the more neural degeneration you have, and the greater your signs of aging. When you take in ketones, your body makes fewer of these oxidants and fights the ones that are already there.

Basically, a ketogenic diet acts like consuming berries on a large scale. Ketones boost the work of glutathione peroxidase, which is part of our built in system that fights oxidants.

Reducing carbohydrate intake also leads to reduced oxidation of glucose (called glycolysis). Because the ketogenic diet is high in fat, it also boosts the polyunsaturated fatty acid levels in the body. Known as PUFAs, these also limit the production of oxidation as well as inflammation.

The stress from inflammation is another threat to your general health, and PUFAs attack the expression of those genes that encode for factors favorable to inflammation.

When your neurons get excited, good things happen. They send signals; process input and allow your brain to function. When they get too excited, though, they are likely to die.

Throughout your life, the brain has to walk a fine line between getting excited and calming down, and they do this using two different neurotransmitter chemicals: GABA (which calms things down) and glutamate (which gets things going). If you tilt more toward excitement, going too far takes you toward such unpleasant destinations as seizures, degenerating neurons and stroke.

The technical term for this is excitotoxicity -- the toxic effects of too much excitement. A study from the 1930s found that injecting ketone bodies directly into rabbits kept chemically induced seizures from happening, because the ketones kept glutamate from releasing.

However, at the time, the researchers could not identify just why this was the case. More recent studies in neurons of the hippocampus showed that ketones kept neurons from taking on too much glutamate.

Another study showed that the ketogenic diet kept mice from losing cells in the hippocampus by inhibiting the molecules that signal those cells to die. In both rodent and human studies, the ketones boost GABA within the synapses (where neurotransmitters emerge). The result of this is a reduction in the incidence of seizure.

If you're looking for more research involving humans rather than animals, a study involving 23 senior citizens with mild cognitive disorders led to significant improvements in verbal memory after a month and a half on a ketogenic diet.

Another study involved 152 patients who suffered from mild to moderate Alzheimer's disease. For three months, the patients either received an agent with ketones or a placebo while staying with their normal diets. The ones getting the ketogenic drug showed significant improvement in comparison to those receiving the placebo.

A pilot study involving seven Parkinson's disease patients had five who could follow the diet for a month. All of them had a significant reduction in the physical signs of the disease.

The most frequent side effects of a ketogenic diet over time appear to include dehydration, constipation and deficiencies in micronutrients and electrolytes.

However, paying attention to hydration often resolves these problems easily. Some patients, usually children, have a higher risk of gallbladder issues, kidney stones and bone fractures. In women, menstrual irregularities can occur, and fertility can suffer as a result. Other than these, no significant side effects have resulted from the ketogenic diet.

To be sure, the research shows a need for ore large scale clinical trials, controlled by placebos, for patients to see if the ketogenic diet definitely protects the brain. However, the early signs indicate that these protective effects certainly have appeared for some.

For people who are using the ketogenic diet for weight loss purposes, having improvements in brain function would certainly be a bonus. However, you will want to talk to your physician to see if this diet is the right decision for you.

No one should make major nutritional changes without talking to one's doctor beforehand. The upside appears to be tremendous, though, in terms of brain health as well as weight loss.

10: Ketogenic Diet Cooking Tips

Dieting has always been an area of concern for many people, especially in the modern generation. There are various diet plans and recipes used for different purposes including disease treatment and elimination of certain conditions.

Weight loss is one of the common debates of the modern population that is very cautious about any extra pound they put on. Ketogenic diet (KD) is an old plan that has existed for over 90 years and mainly focuses on low carbohydrate intake. This diet is used in treating various diseases and alleviating chronic conditions. It is also a fine diet for reducing body weight.

Here is a detailed description of what Ketogenic diets entail

Ketogenic diet and weight loss

The Ketogenic diet encourages reduction of carbohydrate intake, moderate protein and slightly increase in fat consumption. Carbohydrates are the usual source of fuel/energy used by our body organs like brain and heart.

The carb we take are converted to glucose and carried through the blood streams to body organs where they are burnt for energy. When this intake is reduced, the body will naturally initiate counter mechanisms to maintain a steady supply of energy.

This is done by breaking fat cells into ketone bodies which can be used to substitute glucose molecules. The condition where blood sugar (glucose) level is low and the body is forced to convert its fat into ketone bodies is referred to as ketosis.

There are natural ketosis processes like those resulting from starving and fasting. Using diets to achieve this is often called nutritional ketosis. It occurs when our body mechanisms switch from burning glucose and uses fats as the main source of energy as a result of reduced glucose level and raised ketone bodies.

Our bodies store food in the form of fat cells and deposit them around various locations. This is because proteins and carbohydrates cannot be stored in the body. When there is the risk of excess blood sugar content, normal functioning bodies will convert some of the sugar into fat cells.

This results in unsightly body mass, especially when deposition is concentrated around the belly or flanks. Ketogenic diets subject the body to breaking down these fat cells to produce energy since glucose levels are dropped to insufficient contents.

However, the diet requires a moderate amount of proteins. This is because proteins aid proper digestion and balances metabolism processes. When protein intake is very low, the body may feel starved and this induces reaction processes where available sugar is converted to fat cells. This can lead to food craving and continued accumulation of fat cells which result in weight gain.

Low-carb diets have been preferred in weight loss and Ketogenic in particular has many advantages. Unlike other plans, these diets result in natural breakdown of fat cells which are the main reason for unpleasant weights. This prevents recurrent weight accumulation.

Benefits of Ketogenic Diets

There are several benefits of Ketogenic diet which have been consistently recommended for the past nine decades. This diet does not only aid weight loss, but also reduce blood sugar level making it suitable for various conditions such as diabetes. Ketone bodies and ketosis process are currently under study to determine other potential benefits.

They have been shown to improve overall body metabolism processes. They are also used to control or even eliminate epileptic seizures. Other advantages of this diet include the following;

- Helping Alzheimer's disease patients regain memory
- Reverse heart diseases and PCOC
- Treat severe acne and gluten allergies
- Remiss cancer
- Treat metabolism energy disorders such as GLUT-1

Ketogenic diets require consistency in taking lesser carbohydrates and more natural fats like coconut oil and butter. To fully appreciate the benefits of this diet, one will need to achieve a stable nutritional ketosis.

KD cooking tips

Ketogenic diets cooking is based on avoiding starch and sugars as much as possible and increasing fats and protein intake. All the meals should be made from fresh ingredients and natural fats. This is because processed vegetable fats are known to result in internal inflammation and subsequent complications.

Use low-carb vegetables, salads and sauces to compliment your meal. You should aim at avoiding flour and grains, flour based products such as crackers and bread, starchy vegetables like peas and potatoes as well as sweeteners like corn and sugar syrups.

Traditional techniques that encouraged high amounts of carb like crumbing and breading should be substituted with new low-carb procedures. Avoid processes involving bread crumbs flours and other high carbohydrate contents.

The general cooking processes such as roasting, grilling, steaming, poaching, broiling, sautéing and baking are allowed. However, vegetables can lose some of the vitamins and nutritional value when boiled. Use other methods of cooking to preserve the nutrients or include the stew as part of your meal.

From chicken salads to baked fish, sardines, canned tuna, string cheese, Greek yogurt, and boiled egg, among other low carbohydrate foods, there are many options for ketogenic diets. You can make a quick low-carb ketogenic diet or find an outlet that sells them.

It is important to note that ketosis is never a one time transformation and can take up to 4 weeks to fully a significant ketone level. One can measure their ketone level to determine whether it is sufficient enough to initiate nutritional ketosis which is very critical to weight loss. It is often advisable to go for ketone levels of 0.5 for a stable nutritional ketosis.

Conclusion

Weight loss is very difficult to achieve, particularly since it requires a total transformation of one's diet and other lifestyle habits. The human body has a tendency to quickly initiate counteractive processes to regain the weight that has been lost too fast.

Diets can only produce significant results when they are consistently practiced. As much as low carbohydrates and high fat will initiate natural disintegration of fat cells, moderation is still very necessary.

Overconsumption of proteins and fat will retard the weight loss process. Similarly habits like smoking and excessive drinking may alter metabolism processes and result in unsatisfactory results. Ensure you practice ketogenic diets using fresh ingredients with less sugars and starch for better outcome.

20585424R00040

Made in the USA
Middletown, DE
01 June 2015